The Ultimate Ketogenic Air Fryer Lunch Cooking Guide

A Handful of Quick, Delicious Recipes for Your Ketogenic Air Fryer Meals

Nolan Turner

advice. The content within this book has been derived from various sources. Please consult a licensed professional before attempting any techniques outlined in this book.

By reading this document, the reader agrees that under no circumstances is the author responsible for any losses, direct or indirect, which are incurred as a result of the use of information contained within this document, including, but not limited to, — errors, omissions, or inaccuracies.

5

Table of Contents

Mixed Peppers Hash

Preparation time: 5 minutes **Cooking time:** 20 minutes **Servings:** 4

Ingredients:

1 red bell pepper, cut into strips

green bell pepper, cut into strips 1 orange bell pepper, cut into strips 4 eggs, whisked

Salt and black pepper to the taste

tablespoons mozzarella, shredded Cooking spray

Directions:

In a bowl, mix the eggs with all the bell peppers, salt and pepper and toss. Preheat the air fryer at 350 degrees F, grease it with cooking spray, pour the eggs mixture, spread well, sprinkle the mozzarella on top and cook for 20 minutes. Divide between plates and serve for breakfast.

Nutrition: calories 229, fat 13, fiber 3, carbs 4, protein 7

Baked Eggs

Prep time: 10 minutes **Cooking time:** 10 minutes **Servings:** 3

Ingredients:

3 eggs

½ teaspoon ground turmeric

¼ teaspoon salt

3 bacon slices

1 teaspoon butter, melted

Directions:

Brush the muffin silicone molds with ½ teaspoon of melted butter. Then arrange the bacon in the silicone molds in the shape of circles. Preheat the air fryer to 400F. Cook the bacon for 7 minutes. After this, brush the center of every bacon circle with remaining butter. Then crack the eggs in every bacon circles, sprinkle with salt and ground turmeric. Cook the bacon cups for 3 minutes more.

Nutrition: calories 178, fat 13.6, fiber 0.1, carbs 0.9, protein 12.6

Paprika Cauliflower Bake

Preparation time: 5 minutes **Cooking time:** 20 minutes **Servings:** 4

Ingredients:

2 cups cauliflower florets, separated 4 eggs, whisked

teaspoon sweet paprika

tablespoons butter, melted

A pinch of salt and black pepper

Directions:

Heat up your air fryer at 320 degrees F, grease with the butter, add cauliflower florets on the bottom, then add eggs whisked with paprika, salt and pepper, toss and cook for 20 minutes. Divide between plates and serve for breakfast.

Nutrition: calories 240, fat 9, fiber 2, carbs 4, protein 8

Cinnamon French Toast

Prep time: 12 minutes **Cooking time:** 9 minutes
Servings: 2

Ingredients:

1/3 cup almond flour

1 egg, beaten

¼ teaspoon baking powder

2 teaspoons Erythritol

¼ teaspoon vanilla extract

1 teaspoon cream cheese

¼ teaspoon ground cinnamon

1 teaspoon ghee, melted

Directions:

In the mixing bowl mix up almond flour, baking powder, and ground cinnamon. Then add egg, vanilla extract, ghee, and cream cheese. Stir the mixture with the help of the fork until homogenous. Line the mugs bottom with baking paper. After this, transfer the almond flour mixture in the mugs and flatten well. Then preheat the air fryer to 355F. Place the mugs with toasts in the air fryer basket and cook them for 9 minutes. When the time is finished and the toasts are cooked, cool them little. Then sprinkle the toasts with Erythritol.

Nutrition: calories 85, fat 7.2, fiber 0.7, carbs 1.8, protein 3.9

Cheddar Tomatoes Hash

Preparation time: 5 minutes **Cooking time:** 25 minutes **Servings:** 4

Ingredients:

2 tablespoons olive oil

pound tomatoes, chopped

½ pound cheddar, shredded

tablespoons chives, chopped Salt and black pepper to the taste 6 eggs, whisked

Directions:

Add the oil to your air fryer, heat it up at 350 degrees F, add the tomatoes, eggs, salt and pepper and whisk. Also add the cheese on top and sprinkle the chives on top. Cook for 25 minutes, divide between plates and serve for breakfast.

Nutrition: calories 221, fat 8, fiber 3, carbs 4, protein 8

Scotch Eggs

Prep time: 15 minutes **Cooking time:** 13 minutes
Servings: 4

Ingredients:

4 medium eggs, hard-boiled, peeled

9 oz ground beef

1 teaspoon garlic powder

¼ teaspoon cayenne pepper

1 oz coconut flakes

¼ teaspoon curry powder

1 egg, beaten

1 tablespoon almond·flour

Cheesy Frittata

Preparation time: 10 minutes **Cooking time:** 20 minutes **Servings:** 6

Ingredients:

1 cup almond milk Cooking spray

9 ounces cream cheese, soft

1 cup cheddar cheese, shredded 6 spring onions, chopped

Salt and black pepper to the taste 6 eggs, whisked

Directions:

Heat up your air fryer with the oil at 350 degrees F and grease it with cooking spray. In a bowl, mix the eggs with the rest of the ingredients, whisk well, pour and spread into the air fryer and cook everything for 20 minutes. Divide everything between plates and serve.

Nutrition: calories 231, fat 11, fiber 3, carbs 5, protein 8

Eggs Ramekins

Prep time: 5 minutes **Cooking time:** 6 minutes
Servings: 5

Ingredients:

5 eggs

1 teaspoon coconut oil, melted

¼ teaspoon ground black pepper

Directions:

Brush the ramekins with coconut oil and crack the eggs inside. Then sprinkle the eggs with ground black pepper and transfer in the air fryer. Cook the baked eggs for 6 minutes at 355F.

Nutrition: calories 144, fat 8, fiber 4.5, carbs 9.1, protein 8.8

Herbed Omelet

Preparation time: 5 minutes **Cooking time:** 20 minutes **Servings:** 4

Ingredients:

10 eggs, whisked

½ cup cheddar, shredded

2 tablespoons parsley, chopped 2 tablespoons chives, chopped 2 tablespoons basil, chopped Cooking spray

Salt and black pepper to the taste

Directions:

In a bowl, mix the eggs with all the ingredients except the cheese and the cooking spray and whisk well. Preheat the air fryer at 350 degrees F, grease it with the cooking spray, and pour the eggs mixture inside.

Sprinkle the cheese on top and cook for 20 minutes. Divide everything between plates and serve.

Nutrition: calories 232, fat 12, fiber 4, carbs 5, protein 7

Chicken Muffins

Prep time: 10 minutes **Cooking time:** 10 minutes
Servings: 6

Ingredients:

1 cup ground chicken

1 cup ground pork

½ cup Mozzarella, shredded

1 teaspoon dried oregano

½ teaspoon salt

1 teaspoon ground paprika

½ teaspoon white pepper

1 tablespoon ghee, melted

1 teaspoon dried dill

2 tablespoons almond flour

1 egg, beaten

Directions:

In the bowl mix up ground chicken, ground pork, dried oregano, salt, ground paprika, white pepper, dried dill, almond flour, and egg. When you get the homogenous texture of the mass, add ½ of all Mozzarella and mix up the mixture gently with the help of the spoon. Then brush the silicone muffin molds with melted ghee. Put the meat mixture in the muffin molds. Flatten the surface of every muffin with the help of the spoon and top with remaining Mozzarella. Preheat the air fryer to 375F. Then arrange the muffins in the air fryer basket and cook them for 10 minutes. Cool the cooked muffins to the room temperature and remove from the muffin molds.

Nutrition: calories 291, fat 20.6, fiber 1.3, carbs 2.7, protein 23.9

Chives Endives

Preparation time: 5 minutes **Cooking time:** 15 minutes **Servings:** 4

Ingredients:

4 endives, trimmed

A pinch of salt and black pepper

¼ cup goat cheese, crumbled 1 teaspoon lemon zest, grated 1 tablespoon lemon juice

2 tablespoons chives, chopped 2 tablespoons olive oil

Directions:

In a bowl, mix the endives with the other ingredients except the cheese and chives and toss well. Put the endives in your air fryer's basket and cook at 380 degrees F for 15 minutes. Divide the corn between plates and serve with cheese and chives sprinkled on top.

Nutrition: calories 140, fat 4, fiber 3, carbs 5, protein 7

Cheese Zucchini Rolls

Prep time: 20 minutes **Cooking time:** 10 minutes
Servings: 2

Ingredients:

1 large zucchini, trimmed

1 teaspoon keto tomato sauce

3 oz Mozzarella, sliced

1 teaspoon olive oil

Directions:

Slice the zucchini on the long thin slices. Then sprinkle every zucchini slice with marinara sauce and top with sliced Mozzarella. Roll the zucchini and secure it with toothpicks. Preheat the air fryer to 385F. Put the zucchini rolls in the air fryer and sprinkle them with olive oil. Cook the zucchini rolls for 10 minutes.

Nutrition: calories 168, fat 10.2, fiber 1.9, carbs 7.3, protein 14

Endives Sauté

Preparation time: 5 minutes **Cooking time:** 15 minutes **Servings:** 4

Ingredients:

4 endives, trimmed and sliced

A pinch of salt and black pepper 1 tablespoon olive oil

2 shallots, chopped

1 cup white mushrooms, sliced

½ cup parmesan, grated

1 tablespoon parsley, chopped Juice of ½ lemon

Directions:

Heat up a pan that fits the air fryer with the oil over medium-high heat, add the shallots and sauté for 2 minutes. Add the mushrooms, stir and cook for 1-2 minutes more. Add the rest of the ingredients except the parmesan and the parsley, toss, put the pan in the air fryer and cook at 380 degrees F for 10 minutes. Divide everything between plates and serve.

Nutrition: calories 170, fat 4, fiber 3, carbs 5, protein 8

Thyme Mushroom Pan

Prep time: 10 minutes **Cooking time:** 8 minutes
Servings: 2

Ingredients:

1/2 pound cremini mushrooms, sliced

1 cup coconut cream

1 teaspoon avocado oil

¼ teaspoon minced garlic

½ teaspoon dried thyme

Directions:

In the air fryer's pan, mix the mushrooms with the cream
and the other ingredients, toss and cook at 380 degrees
F for 8 minutes. Divide into bowls and serve.

Nutrition: calories 128, fat 5.5, fiber 5, carbs 4.5,
protein 12.8

Parsley Asparagus

Preparation time: 5 minutes **Cooking time:** 15 minutes **Servings:** 4

Ingredients:

pound asparagus, trimmed 1 fennel bulb, quartered

A pinch of salt and black pepper 2 cherry tomatoes, chopped

chili peppers, chopped

2 tablespoons cilantro, chopped 2 tablespoons parsley, chopped 2 tablespoons olive oil

2 tablespoons lemon juice

Directions:

Heat up a pan that fits the air fryer with the oil over medium-high heat, add chili peppers and the fennel and sauté for 2 minutes. Add the rest of the ingredients, toss, put the pan in the air fryer and cook at 380 degrees F for 12 minutes. Divide everything between plates and serve.

Nutrition: calories 163, fat 4, fiber 2, carbs 4, protein 7

Parmesan Spinach Balls

Prep time: 15 minutes **Cooking time:** 5 minutes
Servings: 4

Ingredients:

2 cups spinach, chopped

4 oz Parmesan, grated

½ teaspoon ground nutmeg

½ teaspoon ground black pepper

1 egg, beaten

½ cup coconut flour

1 teaspoon avocado oil

Directions:

Put the spinach in the blender and grind it. Then transfer the grinded spinach in the bowl and mix it up with grated Parmesan, ground nutmeg, ground black pepper, and egg. Stir the mixture carefully and add coconut flour. Mix it up with the help of the spoon. Then make the spinach balls with the help of the fingertips. Preheat the air fryer to 400F. Put the spinach balls in the air fryer and sprinkle with avocado oil. Cook the spinach balls bites for 5 minutes.

Nutrition: calories 184, fat 10, fiber 6.5, carbs 11, protein 14

Collard Greens Sauté

Preparation time: 5 minutes **Cooking time:** 12 minutes **Servings:** 4

Ingredients:

pound collard greens, trimmed

fennel bulbs, trimmed and quartered 2 tablespoons olive oil

Salt and black pepper to the taste

½ cup keto tomato sauce

Directions:

In a pan that fits your air fryer, mix the collard greens with the fennel and the rest of the ingredients, toss, put the pan in the fryer and cook at 350 degrees F for 12 minutes. Divide everything between plates and serve.

Nutrition: calories 163, fat 4, fiber 3, carbs 5, protein 6

Lemon Roasted Peppers

Prep time: 10 minutes **Cooking time:** 8 minutes
Servings: 4

Ingredients:

4 shishito peppers

1 teaspoon lemon juice

½ teaspoon sesame oil

Directions:

Pierce the shishito peppers to make many small cuts and
sprinkle them with lemon juice and sesame oil. Preheat
the air fryer to 400F. Put the peppers in the air fryer
basket and cook them for 4 minutes from each side.

Nutrition: calories 20, fat 0.6, fiber 2, carbs 3, protein
1

Mustard Greens, Green Beans and Sauce

Preparation time: 10 minutes **Cooking time**: 12 minutes **Servings:** 4

Ingredients:

bunch mustard greens, trimmed 1 pound green beans, halved

tablespoons olive oil

¼ cup keto tomato sauce 3 garlic cloves, minced

Salt and black pepper to the taste 1 tablespoon balsamic vinegar

Directions:

In a pan that fits your air fryer, mix the mustard greens with the rest of the ingredients, toss, put the pan in the fryer and cook at 350 degrees F for 12 minutes. Divide everything between plates and serve.

Nutrition: calories 163, fat 4, fiber 3, carbs 4, protein 7

Paprika Green Beans

Preparation time: 5 minutes **Cooking time:** 20 minutes **Servings:** 4

Ingredients:

6 cups green beans, trimmed 2 tablespoons olive oil

1 tablespoon hot paprika

A pinch of salt and black pepper

Directions:

In a bowl, mix the green beans with the other ingredients, toss, put them in the air fryer's basket and cook at 370 degrees F for 20 minutes. Divide between plates and serve as a side dish.

Nutrition: calories 120, fat 5, fiber 1, carbs 4, protein 2

Pecorino Zucchini

Prep time: 15 minutes **Cooking time:** 5 minutes
Servings: 5

Ingredients:

1 large zucchini

2 cherry tomatoes, chopped

1 bell pepper, diced

3 spring onions, diced

1 tablespoon sesame oil

4 oz Pecorino cheese, grated

½ teaspoon chili flakes

¼ teaspoon minced garlic

1 teaspoon flax seeds

Directions:

Make the spirals from the zucchini with the help of the spiralizer and sprinkle with sesame oil. Then place them in the air fryer, add diced bell pepper, and cook for 5 minutes at 355F. After this, transfer the cooked vegetables in the big bowl. Add cherry tomatoes, spring onions, Pecorino, chili flakes, minced garlic, and flax seeds. Mix up zucchini Primavera with the help of 2 spatulas.

Nutrition: calories 169, fat 12.2, fiber 1.9, carbs 6.6, protein 10.7

Smoked Asparagus

Preparation time: 5 minutes **Cooking time:** 20 minutes **Servings:** 4

Ingredients:

pound asparagus stalks

Salt and black pepper to the taste

¼ cup olive oil+ 1 teaspoon 1 tablespoon smoked paprika

tablespoons balsamic vinegar 1 tablespoon lime juice

Directions:

In a bowl, mix the asparagus with salt, pepper and 1 teaspoon oil, toss, transfer to your air fryer's basket and cook at 370 degrees F for 20 minutes. Meanwhile, in a bowl, mix all the other ingredients and whisk them well. Divide the asparagus between plates, drizzle the balsamic vinaigrette all over and serve as a side dish.

Nutrition: calories 187, fat 6, fiber 2, carbs 4, protein 9

Swiss Chard Mix

Prep time: 10 minutes **Cooking time:** 15 minutes
Servings: 5

Ingredients:

7 oz Swiss chard, chopped

4 oz Swiss cheese, grated

4 teaspoons almond flour

½ cup heavy cream

½ teaspoon ground black pepper

Directions:

Mix up Swiss chard and Swiss cheese. Add almond flour, heavy cream, and ground black pepper. Stir the mixture until homogenous. After this, transfer it in 5 small ramekins. Preheat the air fryer to 365F. Place the ramekins with gratin in the air fryer basket and cook them for 15 minutes.

Nutrition: calories 264, fat 22.1, fiber 3.1, carbs 8, protein 11.9

Garlic Lemony Asparagus

Preparation time: 5 minutes **Cooking time:** 15 minutes **Servings:** 4

Ingredients:

1 bunch asparagus, trimmed

Salt and black pepper to the taste 4 tablespoons olive oil

4 garlic cloves, minced Juice of ½ lemon

3 tablespoons parmesan, grated

Directions:

In a bowl, mix the asparagus with all the ingredients except the parmesan, toss, transfer it to your air fryer's basket and cook at 400 degrees F for 15 minutes. Divide between plates, sprinkle the parmesan on top and serve as a side dish.

Nutrition: calories 173, fat 12, fiber 2, carbs 5, protein 7

Hot Broccoli

Prep time: 10 minutes **Cooking time:** 5 minutes
Servings: 4

Ingredients:

11 oz broccoli stems

1 tablespoon olive oil

¼ teaspoon chili powder

Directions:

Preheat the air fryer to 400F. Then chop the broccoli stems roughly and sprinkle with chili powder and olive oil. Transfer the greens in the preheated air fryer and cook them for 5 minutes.

Nutrition: calories 57, fat 3.8, fiber 2.1, carbs 5.3, protein 2.2

Balsamic Greens Sauté

Preparation time: 5 minutes **Cooking time:** 15 minutes **Servings:** 4

Ingredients:

1 pound collard greens

¼ cup cherry tomatoes, halved 1 tablespoon balsamic vinegar A pinch of salt and black pepper 2 tablespoons chicken stock

Directions:

In a pan that fits your air fryer, mix the collard greens with the other ingredients, toss gently, introduce in the air fryer and cook at 360 degrees F for 15 minutes. Divide between plates and serve as a side dish.

Nutrition: calories 121, fat 3, fiber 4, carbs 6, protein 5

Butter Zucchini Noodles

Preparation time: 5 minutes **Cooking time:** 15 minutes **Servings:** 4

Ingredients:

1 pound zucchinis, cut with a spiralizer 2 tomatoes, cubed

3 tablespoons butter, melted 4 garlic cloves, minced

3 tablespoons parsley, chopped Salt and black pepper to the taste

Directions:

In a pan that fits your air fryer, mix all the ingredients, toss, introduce in the fryer and cook at 350 degrees F for 15 minutes. Divide between plates and serve as a side dish.

Nutrition: calories 170, fat 6, fiber 2, carbs 5, protein 6

Dill Bok Choy

Prep time: 20 minutes **Cooking time:** 5 minutes
Servings: 2

Ingredients:

6 oz bok choy

1 teaspoon sesame seeds

1 garlic clove, diced

1 tablespoon olive oil

1 teaspoon fresh dill, chopped

1 teaspoon apple cider vinegar

Directions:

Preheat the air fryer to 350F. Then chop the bok choy roughly and sprinkle with olive oil, diced garlic, olive oil, fresh dill, and apple cider vinegar. Mix up the bok choy and leave to marinate for 15 minutes. Then transfer the marinated bok choy in the air fryer basket and cook for

5 minutes. Shake it after 3 minutes of cooking. Transfer the cooked vegetables in the bowl and sprinkle with sesame seeds. Shake the meal gently before serving.

Nutrition: calories 84, fat 8, fiber 1.1, carbs 3, protein 1.8

Bacon Green Beans Mix

Prep time: 15 minutes **Cooking time:** 13 minutes
Servings: 4

Ingredients:

1 cup green beans, trimmed

4 oz bacon, sliced

¼ teaspoon salt

1 tablespoon avocado oil

Directions:

Wrap the green beans in the sliced bacon. After this, sprinkle the vegetables with salt and avocado oil. Preheat the air fryer to 385F. Carefully arrange the green beans in the air fryer in one layer and cook them for 5 minutes. Then flip the green beans on another side and cook for 8 minutes more.

Nutrition: calories 167, fat 12.3, fiber 0.9, carbs 2.6, protein 10.5

Chicken Wings and Vinegar Sauce

Prep time: 10 minutes **Cooking time:** 12 minutes
Servings: 4

Ingredients:

4 chicken wings

1 teaspoon Erythritol

1 teaspoon water

1 teaspoon apple cider vinegar

1 teaspoon salt

¼ teaspoon ground paprika

½ teaspoon dried oregano

Cooking spray

Directions:

Sprinkle the chicken wings with salt and dried oregano. Then preheat the air fryer to 400F. Place the chicken wings in the air fryer basket and cook them for 8 minutes.

Flip the chicken wings on another side after 4 minutes of cooking. Meanwhile, mix up Erythritol, water, apple cider vinegar, and ground paprika in the saucepan and bring the liquid to boil. Stir the liquid well and cook it until Erythritol is dissolved. After this, generously brush the chicken wings with sweet Erythritol liquid and cook them in the air fryer at 400F for 4 minutes more.

Nutrition: calories 100, fat 6.7, fiber 0.2, carbs 0.3, protein 9.2

Celery Chicken Mix

Prep time: 15 minutes **Cooking time:** 9 minutes **Servings:** 4

Ingredients:

1 teaspoon fennel seeds

½ teaspoon ground celery

½ teaspoon salt

1 tablespoon olive oil

12 oz chicken fillet

Directions:

Cut the chicken fillets on 4 chicken chops. In the shallow bowl mix up fennel seeds and olive oil. Rub the chicken chops with salt and ground celery. Preheat the air fryer to 365F. Brush the chicken chops with the fennel oil and place it in the air fryer basket. Cook them for 9 minutes.

Nutrition: calories 193, fat 9.9, fiber 0.2, carbs 0.3, protein 24.7

Vanilla and Peppercorn Duck

Preparation time: 5 minutes **Cooking time:** 30 minutes **Servings:** 4

Ingredients:

4 duck legs, skin on Juice of ½ lemon

1 teaspoon cinnamon powder 1 teaspoon vanilla extract

10 peppercorns, crushed

1 tablespoon balsamic vinegar 1 tablespoon olive oil

A pinch of salt and black pepper

Directions:

Heat up a pan with the oil over medium-high heat, add the duck legs and sear them for 3 minutes on each side. Transfer to a pan that fits the air fryer, add the remaining ingredients, toss, put the pan in the air fryer and cook at 380 degrees F for 22 minutes. Divide duck legs and cooking juices between plates and serve.

Nutrition: calories 271, fat 13, fiber 4, carbs 6, protein 15

Nutmeg Duck Meatballs

Prep time: 20 minutes **Cooking time:** 10 minutes **Servings:** 6

Ingredients:

1-pound ground duck

½ teaspoon ground cloves

½ teaspoon ground nutmeg

½ teaspoon salt

1 teaspoon dried cilantro

2 tablespoons almond flour

Cooking spray

Directions:

In the mixing bowl mix up ground duck, ground cloves, ground nutmeg, salt, dried cilantro, and almond flour. With the help of the fingertips make the duck meatballs and sprinkle them with cooking spray. Preheat the air fryer to 385F. Put the duck meatballs in the air fryer basket in one layer and cook them for 5 minutes. Then flip the meatballs on another side and cook them for 5 minutes more.

Nutrition: calories 244, fat 16.3, fiber 1.7, carbs 3.4, protein 22.8

Duck with Mushrooms and Coriander

Preparation time: 5 minutes **Cooking time:** 25 minutes **Servings:** 6

Ingredients:

6 duck breasts, boneless, skin on and scored 1 tablespoon balsamic vinegar

1 tablespoon coconut aminos

A pinch of salt and black pepper 2 courgettes, sliced

¼ pound oyster mushrooms, sliced

½ bunch coriander, chopped 2 tablespoons olive oil

garlic cloves, minced

Directions:

Heat up a pan that fits your air fryer with the oil over medium heat, add the duck breasts skin side down and sear for 5 minutes. Add the rest of the ingredients, cook for 2 minutes more, transfer the pan to the air fryer and cook at 380 degrees F for 20 minutes. Divide everything between plates and serve.

Nutrition: calories 2764, fat 12, fiber 4, carbs 6, protein 14

Hot Chicken Skin

Prep time: 10 minutes **Cooking time:** 30 minutes
Servings: 4

Ingredients:

½ teaspoon chili paste

8 oz chicken skin

1 teaspoon sesame oil

½ teaspoon chili powder

½ teaspoon salt

Directions:

In the shallow bowl mix up chili paste, sesame oil, chili powder, and salt. Then brush the chicken skin with chili mixture well and leave for 10 minutes to marinate. Meanwhile, preheat the air fryer to 365F. Put the marinated chicken skin in the air fryer and cook it for 20 minutes. When the time is finished, flip the chicken skin on another side and cook it for 10 minutes more or until the chicken skin is crunchy.

Nutrition: calories 298, fat 25.4, fiber 0.1, carbs 5.7, protein 10.9

Duck with Peppers and Pine Nuts Sauce

Preparation time: 5 minutes **Cooking time:** 25 minutes **Servings:** 4

Ingredients:

duck breast fillets, skin-on

1 tablespoon balsamic vinegar 4 tablespoons olive oil

1 red bell pepper, roasted, peeled and chopped 1/3 cup basil, chopped

1 tablespoon pine nuts 1 teaspoon tarragon

1 garlic clove, minced

1 tablespoon lemon juice

Directions:

Heat up a pan that fist your air fryer with half of the oil over medium heat, add the duck fillets skin side up and cook for 2-3 minutes. Add the vinegar, toss and cook for 2 minutes more. In a blender, combine the rest of the oil with the remaining ingredients and pulse well. Pour this over the duck, put the pan in the fryer and cook at 370 degrees F for 16 minutes.

Divide everything between plates and serve.

Nutrition: calories 270, fat 14, fiber 3, carbs 6, protein 16

Coconut Crusted Chicken

Prep time: 15 minutes **Cooking time:** 9 minutes
Servings: 5

Ingredients:

15 oz chicken fillet

5 eggs, beaten

1 teaspoon salt

½ cup coconut flour

1 teaspoon dried oregano

Cooking spray

Directions:

Cut the chicken fillet on 5 chops and beat them gently with the help of the kitchen hammer. After this, sprinkle the chicken chops with dried oregano and salt. Dip every chicken chop in the beaten eggs and coat in the coconut flour. Preheat the air fryer to 360F. Place the chicken in the air fryer in one layer and cook for 5 minutes. Then flip them on another side and cook for 4 minutes more or until the schnitzels are light brown.

Nutrition: calories 287, fat 12.7, fiber 4.9, carbs 7.7, protein 32.6

Fried Herbed Chicken Wings

Prep time: 10 minutes **Cooking time:** 11 minutes
Servings: 4

Ingredients:

1 tablespoon Emperor herbs chicken spices

8 chicken wings

Cooking spray

Directions:

Generously sprinkle the chicken wings with Emperor herbs chicken spices and place in the preheated to 400F air fryer. Cook the chicken wings for 6 minutes from each side.

Nutrition: calories 220, fat 14.3, fiber 0.6, carbs 3.9, protein 17.7

Duck and Coconut Milk Mix

Preparation time: 5 minutes **Cooking time:** 25 minutes **Servings:** 4

Ingredients:

garlic cloves, minced

duck breasts, boneless, skin-on and scored 2 tablespoons olive oil

¼ teaspoon coriander, ground 14 ounces coconut milk

Salt and black pepper to the taste 1 cup basil, chopped

Directions:

Heat up a pan that fits your air fryer with the oil over medium heat, add the duck breasts, skin side down and sear for 5 minutes. Add the rest of the ingredients, toss, put the pan in the fryer and cook at 380 degrees F for 20 minutes. Divide between plates and serve.

Nutrition: calories 274, fat 13, fiber 3, carbs 5, protein 16

Chia and Hemp Pudding

Prep time: 4 hours **Cooking time:** 2 minutes **Servings:** 2

Ingredients:

1 teaspoon hemp seeds

1 teaspoon chia seeds

1 tablespoon almond flour

1 teaspoon coconut flakes

1 teaspoon walnuts, chopped

½ teaspoon flax meal

¼ teaspoon vanilla extract

½ teaspoon Erythritol

½ cup of coconut milk

¼ cup water, boiled

Directions:

Put hemp seeds, chia seeds, almond flour, coconut flakes, walnuts, flax meal, vanilla extract, coconut milk, and water in the big bowl. Stir the mixture until homogenous and pour it into 2 mason jars. Leave the mason jars in the cold place for 4 hours. Then top the surface of the pudding with Erythritol. Place the mason jars in the air fryer and cook the pudding for 2 minutes at 400F or until you get the light brown crust.

Nutrition: calories 257, fat 24.2, fiber 4.4, carbs 8.4, protein 5.8

Zucchini Salad

Preparation time: 4 minutes **Cooking time:** 15 minutes **Servings:** 2

Ingredients:

cup watercress, torn 1 tablespoon olive oil

cups zucchini, roughly cubed 1 cup parmesan cheese, grated Cooking spray

Directions:

Grease a pan that fits the air fryer with the cooking spray, add all the ingredients except the cheese, sprinkle the cheese on top and cook at 390 degrees F for 15 minutes. Divide into bowls and serve for breakfast.

Nutrition: calories 202, fat 11, fiber 3, carbs 5, protein 4

Sausages Squares

Prep time: 20 minutes **Cooking time:** 20 minutes
Servings: 4

Ingredients:

½ cup almond flour

¼ cup butter, melted

1 egg yolk

½ teaspoon baking powder

¼ teaspoon salt

6 oz sausage meat

¼ teaspoon ground black pepper

Cooking spray

Directions:

Make the dough: in the mixing bowl mix up almond flour,
butter, egg yolk, and baking powder. Add salt and knead
the non-sticky dough. In the separated bowl mix up

ground black pepper and sausage meat. Roll up the dough with the help of the rolling pin. Then cut the dough into squares.

Place the sausage meat in the center of dough squares and secure them in the shape of the puff. Then preheat the air fryer to 320F. Line the air fryer basket with baking paper. Put the sausage puffs over the baking paper and spray them with cooking spray. Cook the meal for 20 minutes at 325F.

Nutrition: calories 280, fat 26.5, fiber 0.4, carbs 1.3, protein 9.8

Tomato and Greens Salad

Preparation time: 5 minutes **Cooking time:** 15 minutes **Servings:** 4

Ingredients:

teaspoon olive oil

cups mustard greens

A pinch of salt and black pepper

½ pound cherry tomatoes, cubed 2 tablespoons chives, chopped

Directions:

Heat up your air fryer with the oil at 360 degrees F, add all the ingredients, toss, cook for 15 minutes shaking halfway, divide into bowls and serve for breakfast.

Nutrition: calories 224, fat 8, fiber 2, carbs 3, protein 7

Cabbage and Pork Hash

Prep time: 15 minutes **Cooking time:** 20 minutes **Servings:** 4

Ingredients:

1 Chinese cabbage, shredded

¼ cup chicken broth

½ teaspoon keto tomato sauce

1 green bell pepper, chopped

1 teaspoon salt

6 oz pork loin, chopped

1 tablespoon apple cider vinegar

1 teaspoon sesame oil

½ teaspoon chili flakes

½ teaspoon salt

¼ teaspoon ground black pepper

1 teaspoon ground turmeric

Directions:

Put Chinese cabbage in the bowl. Add chicken broth, tomato sauce, bell pepper, and salt. Mix up the ingredients and transfer in the air fryer basket. Cook the cabbage for 5 minutes at 365F. Meanwhile, in the mixing bowl mix up ground black pepper, turmeric, salt, chili flakes, sesame oil, and apple cider vinegar. Add chopped pork loin and mix up the ingredients. Add the meat in the air fryer and cook the cabbage hash for 10 minutes at 385F. Then shake the hash well and cook it for 5 minutes more.

Nutrition: calories 131, fat 7.3, fiber 0.8, carbs 3.3, protein 12.6

Green Beans Salad

Preparation time: 5 minutes **Cooking time:** 15 minutes **Servings:** 4

Ingredients:

1 and ¾ cups radishes, chopped

½ pound green beans, trimmed A pinch of salt and black pepper 4 eggs, whisked

Cooking spray

1 tablespoon cilantro, chopped

Directions:

Grease a pan that fits the air fryer with the cooking spray, add all the ingredients, toss and cook at 360 degrees F for 15 minutes. Divide between plates and serve for breakfast.

Nutrition: calories 212, fat 12, fiber 3, carbs 4, protein 9

Coriander Sausages Muffins

Prep time: 10 minutes **Cooking time:** 12 minutes
Servings: 4

Ingredients:

4 teaspoons coconut flour

1 tablespoon coconut cream

1 egg, beaten

½ teaspoon baking powder

6 oz sausage meat

1 teaspoon spring onions, chopped

½ teaspoon ground coriander

1 teaspoon sesame oil

½ teaspoon salt

Directions:

In the mixing bowl mix up coconut flour, coconut cream, egg, baking powder, minced onion, and ground coriander. Add salt and whisk the mixture until smooth. After this, add the sausage meat and stir the muffin batter. Preheat the air fryer to 385F. Brush the muffin molds with sesame oil and pour the batter inside. Place the rack in the air fryer basket. Put the muffins on a rack. Cook the meal for 12 minutes.

Nutrition: calories 239, fat 17.2, fiber 5.1, carbs 8.7, protein 11.7

Cauliflower Rice and Spinach Mix

Preparation time: 5 minutes **Cooking time:** 15 minutes **Servings:** 4

Ingredients:

12 ounces cauliflower rice 3 tablespoons stevia

2 tablespoons olive oil 2 tablespoons lime juice

pound fresh spinach, torn 1 red bell pepper, chopped

Directions:

In your air fryer, mix all the ingredients, toss, cook at 370 degrees F for 15 minutes, shaking halfway, divide between plates and serve for breakfast.

Nutrition: calories 219, fat 14, fiber 3, carbs 5, protein 7

Cheesy Sausage Sticks

Prep time: 15 minutes **Cooking time:** 8 minutes
Servings: 3

Ingredients:

6 small pork sausages

½ cup almond flour

½ cup Mozzarella cheese, shredded

2 eggs, beaten

1 tablespoon mascarpone

Cooking spray

Directions:

Pierce the hot dogs with wooden coffee sticks to get the sausages on the sticks". Then in the bowl mix up almond flour, Mozzarella cheese, and mascarpone. Microwave the mixture for 15 seconds or until you get a melted mixture. Then stir the egg in the cheese mixture and whisk it until smooth. Coat every sausage stick in the cheese mixture. Then preheat the air fryer to 375F. Spray the air fryer basket with cooking spray. Place the sausage stock in the air fryer and cook them for 4 minutes from each side or until they are light brown.

Nutrition: calories 375, fat 32.2, fiber 0.5, carbs 5.1, protein 16.3

Avocado and Cabbage Salad

Preparation time: 5 minutes **Cooking time:** 15 minutes **Servings:** 4

Ingredients:

cups red cabbage, shredded A drizzle of olive oil

1 red bell pepper, sliced

small avocado, peeled, pitted and sliced Salt and black pepper to the taste

Directions:

Grease your air fryer with the oil, add all the ingredients, toss, cover and cook at 400 degrees F for 15 minutes. Divide into bowls and serve cold for breakfast.

Nutrition: calories 209, fat 8, fiber 2, carbs 4, protein 9

Lemon and Almond Cookies

Prep time: 10 minutes **Cooking time:** 8 minutes
Servings: 4

Ingredients:

4 tablespoons coconut flour

½ teaspoon baking powder

1 teaspoon lemon juice

¼ teaspoon vanilla extract

¼ teaspoon lemon zest, grated

2 eggs, beaten

¼ cup of organic almond milk

1 teaspoon avocado oil

¼ teaspoon Himalayan pink salt

Directions:

In the big bowl mix up all ingredients from the list above. Knead the soft dough and cut it into 4 pieces. Preheat the air fryer to 400F. Then line the air fryer basket with baking paper. Roll the dough pieces in the balls and press them gently to get the shape of flat cookies. Place the cookies in the air fryer and cook them for 8 minutes.

Nutrition: calories 74, fat 3.8, fiber 3.1, carbs 5.6, protein 4.4

Turkey and Leeks

Preparation time: 5 minutes **Cooking time:** 30 minutes **Servings:** 4

Ingredients:

1 turkey breast, skinless, boneless and cut into strips A pinch of salt and black pepper

1 tablespoon olive oil 1 cup veggie stock

4 leeks, sliced

2 tablespoon chives, chopped

Directions:

Heat up a pan that fits your air fryer with the oil over medium heat, add the meat and brown for 2 minutes on each side. Add the remaining ingredients, toss, put the pan in the machine and cook at 380 degrees F for 25 minutes. Divide everything between plates and serve with a side salad.

Nutrition: calories 257, fat 12, fiber 4, carbs 5, protein 14

Cumin Turkey and Celery

Preparation time: 5 minutes **Cooking time:** 30 minutes **Servings:** 4

Ingredients:

1 big turkey breast, skinless, boneless and sliced 4 garlic cloves, minced

tablespoons olive oil

celery stalks, roughly chopped 1 teaspoon turmeric powder

1 teaspoon cumin, ground

1 tablespoon smoked paprika 1 tablespoon garlic powder

Directions:

In a pan that fits the air fryer, combine the turkey and the other ingredients, toss, put the pan in the machine and cook at 380 degrees F for 30 minutes. Divide everything between plates and serve.

Nutrition: calories 285, fat 12, fiber 3, carbs 6, protein 16

Chicken Pockets

Prep time: 15 minutes **Cooking time:** 4 minutes
Servings: 4

Ingredients:

2 low carb tortillas

2 oz Cheddar cheese, grated

1 tomato, chopped

1 teaspoon fresh cilantro, chopped

½ teaspoon dried basil

2 teaspoons butter

6 oz chicken fillet, boiled

1 teaspoon sunflower oil

½ teaspoon salt

Directions:

Cut the tortillas into halves. Shred the chicken fillet with the help of the fork and put it in the bowl. Add chopped tomato, grated cheese, basil, cilantro, and alt. Then grease the tortilla halves with butter from one side. Put the shredded chicken mixture on half of every tortilla piece and fold them into the pockets. Preheat the air fryer to 400F. Brush every tortilla pocket with sunflower oil and put it in the air fryer. Cook the meal for 4 minutes.

Nutrition: calories 208, fat 12, fiber 3.7, carbs 6.8, protein 17.5

Buttery Turkey and Mushroom Sauce

Preparation time: 5 minutes **Cooking time:** 25 minutes **Servings:** 4

Ingredients:

6 cups leftover turkey meat, skinless, boneless and shredded A pinch of salt and black pepper

1 tablespoon parsley, chopped 1 cup chicken stock

3 tablespoons butter, melted 1 pound mushrooms, sliced

2 spring onions, chopped

Directions:

Heat up a pan that fits the air fryer with the butter over medium-high heat, add the mushrooms and sauté for 5 minutes. Add the rest of the ingredients, toss, put the pan in the machine and cook at 370 degrees F for 20 minutes. Divide everything between plates and serve.

Nutrition: calories 285, fat 11, fiber 3, carbs 5, protein 14

Ricotta and Thyme Chicken

Prep time: 15 minutes **Cooking time:** 18 minutes
Servings: 3

Ingredients:

3 chicken thighs, boneless

2 teaspoons adobo sauce

1 teaspoon ricotta cheese

1 teaspoon dried thyme

Cooking spray

Directions:

In the mixing bowl mix up adobo sauce and ricotta cheese, Add dried thyme and churn the mixture. Then brush the chicken thighs with adobo sauce mixture and leave for 10 minutes to marinate. Preheat the air fryer to 385F. Spray the air fryer basket with cooking spray and put the chicken thighs inside. Cook them for 18 minutes.

Nutrition: calories 138, fat 7.2, fiber 0.1, carbs 1.4, protein 19.2

Coconut Turkey and Spinach Mix

Preparation time: 5 minutes **Cooking time:** 15 minutes **Servings:** 4

Ingredients:

1 pound turkey meat, ground and browned 1 tablespoon garlic, minced

tablespoon ginger, grated

tablespoons coconut aminos 4 cups spinach leaves

A pinch of salt and black pepper

Directions:

In a pan that fits your air fryer, combine all the ingredients and toss. Put the pan in the air fryer and cook at 380 degrees F for 15 minutes Divide everything into bowls and serve.

Nutrition: calories 240, fat 12, fiber 3, carbs 5, protein 13

Spicy Thyme Chicken Breast

Prep time: 10 minutes **Cooking time:** 17 minutes
Servings: 3

Ingredients:

1-pound chicken breast, skinless, boneless

1 teaspoon garlic powder

1 teaspoon dried thyme

1 teaspoon salt

½ teaspoon ground black pepper

½ teaspoon cayenne pepper

2 teaspoons sunflower oil

Directions:

Sprinkle the chicken breast with garlic powder, dried thyme, salt, ground black pepper, and cayenne pepper. Then gently brush the chicken with sunflower oil and put it in the air fryer. Cook the chicken breast for 17 minutes at 385F. Slice the cooked chicken into servings.

Nutrition: calories 206, fat 7, fiber 0.4, carbs 1.3, protein 32.3

Garlic Turkey and Lemon Asparagus

Preparation time: 5 minutes **Cooking time:** 25 minutes **Servings:** 4

Ingredients:

1 pound turkey breast tenderloins, cut into strips

1 pound asparagus, trimmed and cut into medium pieces
A pinch of salt and black pepper

1 tablespoon lemon juice

teaspoon coconut aminos 2 tablespoons olive oil

garlic cloves, minced

¼ cup chicken stock

Directions:

Heat up a pan that fits the air fryer with the oil over medium-high heat, add the meat and brown for 2 minutes on each side. Add the rest of the ingredients, toss, put the pan in the machine and cook at 380 degrees

F for 20 minutes. Divide everything between plates and serve

Nutrition: calories 264, fat 14, fiber 4, carbs 6, protein 16